FLUCON/

MW01206009

The Medical Book On Fluconazole Guide To Treat Various Fungal Infections

DR. JOHN ANDERSON

Fluconazole, a stalwart in the pharmacological arsenal, stands as a beacon in the realm of antifungal medications. Its advent marked a significant leap forward in the treatment of various fungal infections, offering a potent and versatile therapeutic option. This azole antifungal agent, discovered in the late 1970s, has since become a cornerstone in the management of candidiasis, cryptococcal meningitis, and other fungal maladies. Its mechanism of action, pharmacokinetic profile, and spectrum of activity have solidified its status as a frontline therapy, demonstrating efficacy across a broad spectrum of fungal pathogens. In this introduction, we delve into the multifaceted facets of fluconazole, exploring its pharmacology, clinical applications, adverse effects, and emerging trends in antifungal therapy. Join us as we embark on a journey through the captivating landscape of fluconazole, unraveling its mysteries and uncovering its enduring significance in modern medicine.

FLUCONAZOLE MECHANISM

Fluconazole, a member of the azole class of antifungal medications, exerts its therapeutic effects by interfering with the synthesis of ergosterol, a vital component of fungal cell membranes. This disruption compromises the integrity and function of the fungal cell, ultimately leading to its death.

Here's a step-by-step explanation of the mechanism of fluconazole:

1. **Inhibition of Lanosterol 14-Alpha-Demethylase**: Fluconazole works by inhibiting the enzyme lanosterol 14-alpha-demethylase, which is essential for the synthesis of ergosterol. This enzyme is encoded

by the ERG11 gene in fungi. By inhibiting lanosterol 14-alpha-demethylase, fluconazole prevents the conversion of lanosterol, a precursor molecule, into ergosterol, the final product in the pathway.

2. **Disruption of Ergosterol Synthesis**: Ergosterol is a critical component of fungal cell membranes, providing structural support and regulating membrane fluidity. Without adequate ergosterol, the fungal cell membrane becomes structurally unstable and more permeable.

3. **Accumulation of Abnormal Sterols**: Inhibition of lanosterol 14-alpha-demethylase by fluconazole leads to the accumulation of intermediate sterol compounds, such as 14-alpha-methyl-ergosta-8,24(28)-dien-3beta,6alpha-diol. These abnormal sterols disrupt membrane function and contribute to the destabilization of the fungal cell membrane.

4. **Cellular Dysfunction and Death**: The disruption of ergosterol synthesis and accumulation of abnormal sterols impair vital cellular processes, including nutrient uptake, cell signaling, and membrane

transport. As a result, fungal cells are unable to maintain homeostasis and undergo dysfunction, leading to cell death.

Importantly, fluconazole exhibits selective toxicity towards fungal cells while sparing human cells. This selectivity is attributed to differences in the composition of cell membranes between fungi and humans. While fungal cells rely on ergosterol for membrane integrity, human cells utilize cholesterol. Therefore, fluconazole's action on ergosterol synthesis has minimal impact on human cells, reducing the risk of toxicity.

Overall, fluconazole's mechanism of action involves inhibition of lanosterol 14-alpha-demethylase, disruption of ergosterol synthesis, accumulation of abnormal sterols, and subsequent cellular dysfunction, ultimately leading to fungal cell death. This mechanism underlies the efficacy of fluconazole in treating a wide range of fungal infections.

HISTORY OF FLUCONAZOLE

The history of fluconazole traces back to the late 1970s when researchers at Pfizer were exploring potential antifungal agents. In 1979, fluconazole was discovered as part of this research effort. It was synthesized by chemists Bruce Roth and Robert Vazquez and initially known as UK-49,858.

Initially, fluconazole was primarily investigated for its antifungal properties and its potential to treat a range of fungal infections. Early studies demonstrated its potent activity against various fungal pathogens, including Candida species and Cryptococcus neoformans.

In 1988, fluconazole received approval from the United States Food and Drug Administration (FDA) for the treatment of vaginal candidiasis, marking its first clinical indication. This approval was a significant milestone, as fluconazole became the first systemic antifungal medication available in oral form for the treatment of vaginal yeast infections.

Over the following years, fluconazole's clinical applications expanded as further research demonstrated its efficacy in treating other fungal infections, including oropharyngeal candidiasis, esophageal candidiasis, systemic candidiasis, and cryptococcal meningitis.

One of the key advantages of fluconazole is its excellent bioavailability, allowing for both oral and intravenous administration. This versatility has made it a valuable tool in the management of fungal infections, particularly in hospitalized patients where intravenous therapy may be necessary.

Fluconazole's safety profile and efficacy have led to its widespread use as a first-line treatment for many fungal infections. It is considered a cornerstone of antifungal therapy and is included in treatment guidelines worldwide.

Beyond its clinical applications, fluconazole has also been studied for its potential in prophylactic use, particularly in immunocompromised patients at risk of fungal infections. Additionally, research continues to explore novel formulations and drug delivery systems to enhance its effectiveness and minimize adverse effects.

DOSAGE GUIDE

The dosage of fluconazole can vary depending on the type and severity of the fungal infection being treated, as well as individual patient factors such as age, weight, and overall health. It's crucial to follow the prescribed dosage and administration instructions provided by a healthcare professional. Below is a general guide to the dosage of fluconazole for common fungal infections:

1. **Vaginal Candidiasis**:

   - For uncomplicated infections: A single oral dose of 150 mg is often sufficient.

   - For recurrent infections: A regimen of 150 mg once weekly for 6 months may be prescribed.

2. **Oropharyngeal and Esophageal Candidiasis**:

- Initial treatment: Typically, a loading dose of 200 mg on the first day, followed by 100 to 200 mg once daily for 7 to 14 days.

- Severe infections or immunocompromised patients may require higher doses.

3. **Systemic Candidiasis**:

- Initial treatment: A loading dose of 800 mg on the first day, followed by 400 mg once daily.

- Duration of therapy depends on the response to treatment and the severity of the infection.

4. **Cryptococcal Meningitis**:

- Induction therapy: A loading dose of 800 mg on the first day, followed by 400 to 800 mg once daily for 10 to 12 weeks.

- Maintenance therapy: 200 to 400 mg once daily may be continued indefinitely to prevent relapse in patients with HIV/AIDS.

5. **Prophylaxis of Candidiasis in Immunocompromised Patients**:

- Generally, a dose of 100 to 200 mg once daily may be used, depending on the individual's risk factors and the underlying condition.

It's important to note that dosages may need adjustment in patients with impaired renal function, hepatic impairment, or other medical conditions. Additionally, fluconazole may interact with certain medications, so it's essential to inform the healthcare provider about all medications, supplements, and medical conditions before starting treatment.

This dosage guide provides a general overview, but specific dosing should be determined by a healthcare professional based on individual circumstances and the latest clinical guidelines. Always adhere to the prescribed dosage and duration of treatment for optimal effectiveness and safety.

SIDE EFFECTS

Certainly, fluconazole, like any medication, can cause side effects. While many people tolerate it well, some individuals may experience adverse reactions. Here's a detailed breakdown of potential side effects associated with fluconazole:

1. **Gastrointestinal Disturbances**: Nausea, vomiting, diarrhea, and abdominal pain are common side effects. These symptoms are usually mild and transient. Taking fluconazole with food may help alleviate gastrointestinal discomfort.

2. **Headache**: Some individuals may experience headaches while taking fluconazole. These headaches are typically mild and may resolve with continued use.

3. **Skin Reactions**: Skin rash, itching, and hives can occur as allergic reactions to fluconazole. These reactions may vary in severity, with mild itching to severe rashes. Serious skin reactions such as Stevens-Johnson syndrome or toxic epidermal necrolysis are rare but require immediate medical attention.

4. **Liver Function Abnormalities**: Fluconazole can occasionally lead to changes in liver function tests, manifesting as elevated liver enzymes. Liver function should be monitored, especially in individuals with pre-existing liver conditions or

those taking other medications known to affect the liver.

5. **Hematological Changes**: Fluconazole may cause alterations in blood cell counts, including decreased white blood cell count (neutropenia), decreased platelet count (thrombocytopenia), and decreased red blood cell count (anemia). Regular blood tests may be necessary to monitor for these changes.

6. **Central Nervous System Effects**: Rarely, fluconazole may cause central nervous system side effects such as dizziness, seizures, or

hallucinations. These side effects are more likely to occur in individuals with underlying neurological conditions.

7. **Allergic Reactions**: Some people may experience allergic reactions to fluconazole, including swelling of the face, lips, or tongue; difficulty breathing; or severe dizziness. Anaphylaxis, while rare, is a severe allergic reaction that requires immediate medical attention.

8. **Others**: Other less common side effects of fluconazole may

include taste disturbances, hair loss, fatigue, and photosensitivity (increased sensitivity to sunlight).

It's essential to be aware of these potential side effects and to promptly report any unusual or severe symptoms to a healthcare professional. In most cases, side effects are manageable, and healthcare providers can provide guidance on how to alleviate symptoms or adjust treatment if necessary.

PRECAUTIONS

When using fluconazole, it's important to take certain precautions to ensure safe and effective treatment. Here are some precautions to consider:

1. **Medical History**: Inform your healthcare provider about your complete medical history, including any allergies, liver or kidney problems, heart conditions, or other medical conditions you may have. This information can help determine if fluconazole is the right medication for you and if any dose adjustments are necessary.

2. **Medication Interactions**: Inform your healthcare provider about all the medications you are currently taking, including prescription drugs, over-the-counter medications, supplements, and herbal remedies. Some medications can interact with fluconazole, potentially affecting its effectiveness or increasing the risk of side effects.

3. **Pregnancy and Breastfeeding**: If you are pregnant, planning to become pregnant, or breastfeeding, discuss the risks and benefits of using fluconazole with your healthcare provider. While fluconazole is generally considered safe during

pregnancy, it may be associated with a slightly higher risk of birth defects when used in high doses during the first trimester. Your healthcare provider can help weigh the potential risks and benefits and determine the most appropriate course of action.

4. **Liver and Kidney Function**: Since fluconazole is primarily metabolized by the liver and excreted by the kidneys, it's important to monitor liver and kidney function regularly, especially in individuals with pre-existing liver or kidney conditions. Your healthcare provider may adjust the dosage of fluconazole

based on your liver and kidney function tests.

5. **Alcohol**: Avoid consuming alcohol while taking fluconazole, as it can increase the risk of liver toxicity and other side effects.

6. **Driving and Operating Machinery**: Some people may experience dizziness or other central nervous system side effects while taking fluconazole. If you experience these side effects, avoid driving or operating machinery until you know how the medication affects you.

7. **Sun Exposure**: Fluconazole may increase sensitivity to sunlight (photosensitivity) in some individuals. Use sunscreen and protective clothing when outdoors to reduce the risk of sunburn.

8. **Completion of Treatment**: Take fluconazole for the full prescribed duration, even if your symptoms improve before the medication is finished. Skipping doses or stopping treatment prematurely can lead to incomplete eradication of the infection and potential recurrence.

Always follow the instructions provided by your healthcare provider and read the medication label carefully. If you have any questions or concerns about using fluconazole, don't hesitate to consult with your healthcare provider for personalized guidance and advice.

Made in United States
Troutdale, OR
09/20/2024

23006379R00018